YOUR KNOWLEDGE HAS VALUE

- We will publish your bachelor's and master's thesis, essays and papers

- Your own eBook and book - sold worldwide in all relevant shops

- Earn money with each sale

Upload your text at www.GRIN.com
and publish for free

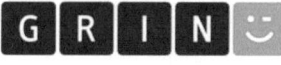

Bibliographic information published by the German National Library:

The German National Library lists this publication in the National Bibliography; detailed bibliographic data are available on the Internet at http://dnb.dnb.de .

This book is copyright material and must not be copied, reproduced, transferred, distributed, leased, licensed or publicly performed or used in any way except as specifically permitted in writing by the publishers, as allowed under the terms and conditions under which it was purchased or as strictly permitted by applicable copyright law. Any unauthorized distribution or use of this text may be a direct infringement of the author s and publisher s rights and those responsible may be liable in law accordingly.

Imprint:

Copyright © 2018 GRIN Verlag
Print and binding: Books on Demand GmbH, Norderstedt Germany
ISBN: 9783668749856

This book at GRIN:

https://www.grin.com/document/428608

Patrick Kimuyu

Sociology of the Body. Forms of "Body" and its Connection to Health Issues

GRIN - Your knowledge has value

Since its foundation in 1998, GRIN has specialized in publishing academic texts by students, college teachers and other academics as e-book and printed book. The website www.grin.com is an ideal platform for presenting term papers, final papers, scientific essays, dissertations and specialist books.

Visit us on the internet:

http://www.grin.com/

http://www.facebook.com/grincom

http://www.twitter.com/grin_com

Table of Contents

Introduction 1
Theorizing Bodies 1
    The Physical Body 2
    The Personal Body 3
    The Expressive Body 3
    The Knowledgeable Body 3
    The Political Body 4
The Body in Symbolic Interaction 4
    Body as Performance: The Dramaturgical Body 4
    Reflexivity as Embodiment: The Looking-Glass Body 5
    Body as Province of Meaning: The Phenomenological Body 5
    Body as Story: The Narrative Body 5
    Body as Trace of Culture: The Socio-Semiotic Body 6
Sociology of Health, Illness and Sexuality 6
Conclusion 7
References 8

Introduction

Sociology seems to have undergone a series of revolution to advance the scope of human nature, especially with regard to philosophies and human understanding of the social aspect of mankind. In general, sociology is one of the disciplines regarded to as social sciences but, it emerged after psychology, economics and anthropology had been studied extensively. However, these disciplines could not address the human's social nature satisfactorily, especially during the revolutionary moments, in Europe in 18th and 19th centuries. Modernists trace back the emergence of sociology to the French Revolution of 1787 and, the discipline is believed to have favored by the Industrial Revolution of the 19th century, owing to the transient changes in social life (Low & Malacrida, 2008). New aspects such as capitalism, democracy and individualism defined social life as a unique feature of mankind.

Since its inception, sociology has been changing to assume diverse forms. For instance, Sociology of the Body emerged recently as one of the fundamental branches of Sociology. Historically, Sociology was viewed on cultural and societal perspectives, and the body was considered as a peripheral element in the discipline. Shilling (2003) remarks, "the body has historically been something of an 'absent presence' in sociology (p. 17). Moreover, Waskul and Vannini (2005) reiterate Anthony Synnott's remarks, "we can usefully reconsider the body at the heart of sociology, rather than peripheral to the discipline, and more importantly at the heart of our social lives and our sense of self" (p. 1).

In Sociology of the body, the body is considered as an interplay of multiple manifestations, identities, hierarchies and relations and, Kelland (2006) remarks, "That interplay results in an individual's unique way of knowing, their personal epistemology" (p. 215). Therefore, this research paper will give a comprehensive overview on the core elements of the Sociology of the Body. It will digress into the principal tenets of the discipline and, discuss how the human body has been theorized to address different roles. It will also discuss the role of the body in symbolic interaction and the sociology of health.

Theorizing Bodies

In regard to the Sociology of the Body, the physical or rather the biological body can be represented in diverse ways, through which the roles of the body's social element can be explained. Ordinarily, sociologists viewed the social nature of human beings with respect to the manifestations of the mind but, phenomenological approaches have led to the theorizing of the body in various ways. The body has been theorized into physical, personal, expressive, knowledgeable and political bodies.

The Physical Body

From a phenomenal perspective, the physical body is composed of the biological components such as the cells and the nerves. The interaction of the biological components of the body with the environment is believed to play a pivotal role in constructing knowledge and experience. The body recognizes the environment through senses, which enables it to gather information from the ambient environment and, generate experiences; thus, intellectual or practical knowledge is believed to be the product of the body. As such, the body serves as an instrument for the acquisition of all external knowledge (Kelland, 2006). The second role of the body is to coordinate the internal and external environments, in which it gathers information from the external environment through senses. It can synthesize information acquired through listening to speeches or visualizing of physical objects; thus, the body acts as a significant interface between the external and internal environments of an individual. Kelland (2006) states that, "It is through the acquisition of sensory information, considered in the context of previous knowledge that the learner constructs a [more] complete understanding of the world" (p. 216). Therefore, the construction of knowledge and real life experiences can be attributed to the physical body.

From another perspective, the body and the mind are believed to be intertwined, unlike in the past when an accentuated divide existed leading to the notion that the mind was responsible for all the social aspects of human beings. The aspects of knowledge acquisition, performing different actions and the status of being of the body and the mind enhance efficient interaction between individuals and the environment, and this embeds nature with a magnificent feature. Therefore, the body plays a significant role in knowledge acquisition; thus, it is instrumental in understanding the circulating discourses. The body and the mind are interactive in a manner, which manifests unification between the two because; the body is inflected into the mind and mind into the body in a unique inversion (Kelland, 2006). Concisely, bodies are useful in manipulating objects and the synthesis of ideas from the mind; thus, the physical body plays significant roles in generating senses, movement and the acquisition of new knowledge from the environment, especially in the form of experiences.

The Personal Body

On the other hand, the personal body defines personal identity and individuality because; body surface and extremities mark its boundaries, separating individuals as distinct entities (Heim 2001). It is believed that the physical boundaries of the body manifest its presence as a solid form to be acknowledged. However, it is worth noting that the boundaries of the body can be established in diverse ways. Kelland (2006) states that, "There are boundaries of the body that are established through dieting, cosmetic surgery, and posture, which 'discipline' the body to be seen as a limitation, rather than a space for expression" (p. 216). In regard to gender, men's' body serves as a means of exploration, whereas the female body is perceived as an enclosure. Therefore, the physical process can be used in establishing limits and boundaries of the personal body, although social inculcation can defines individuality, more or less the same way as the physical process.

The Expressive Body

The body is also believed to be a significant instrument for communication and interpersonal interaction. It is in the body where emotions are generated and expressed. In most cases, emotional reactions determine the interaction between individuals, which are manifested as verbal communication. Physical contact is also believed to be a reliable mode of communication between individuals; thus, self-expression occurs in different ways.

The Knowledgeable Body

Fourthly, the body serves as storage for information, in which knowledge is stored in the mind. On the other hand, the body plays a significant role in transforming knowledge into skills. Transformation of knowledge into skills is manifested by the physical activities of the body. Kelland (2006) states that, "individuals have knowledge, information and experiences that are stored within the body and the mind, and whose presence and origins may be outside their everyday awareness" (p. 218). It is believed that physical skills and tactical memory are stored in the body for tacit understanding. As a result, knowledge stored within the bodies of different individuals can only be expressed in diverse ways with regard to the uniqueness of the stored information. However, it is worth noting that physical skills can only be expressed by individuals who possess appropriate features to communicate the knowledge; thus, knowledge appears to be a significant embodiment in individuals. This aspect enables individuals to undertake various activities in their day-to-day life, especially within organizations because; the individuals' bodies are filled with knowledge.

The Political Body

Inscription manifests the political body, in which an individual's identity is defined with regard to culture, gender and race. As a result, political relationship among groups and individuals can be explored with regard to the body and, the involvement of technologies distinguishes bodies as maps of power and identity (Haraway, 2001). Concisely, modern sociologists believe that human perception and understanding of the environment is attributed to the body. Therefore, bodies, which do not manifest appropriate norms, are excluded in the ecosystem; thus, the body can be theorized as the political body.

The Body in Symbolic Interaction

From a phenomenal perspective, the body is can be regarded to as a subject and object because; it serves as a symbol of self and it also defines an individual. Therefore, experiences of embodiment are usually related to the body. In general, the body plays a pivotal role in symbolic interaction. It is used in performance, narration, embodiment and the interpretation of expressions. It also serves as trace of culture. Some sociologists believe that the body serves as a significant instrument, which defines personhood and society (Waskul & Vannini, 2005).

Body as Performance: The Dramaturgical Body

The dramaturgical body is believed to emphasize on human agency, especially with regard to the analytical and the conceptual framework. In most cases, social and cultural rituals produce experiences of embodiment among individuals in the society. This is so because; rituals are practised at both personal and communal levels. Waskul and Vannini (2005) state, "In our society the character one performs and one's self are somewhat equated and this self-as-character is usually seen as something housed within the body of its possessor" (p. 6).

In the cultural dances, the body performs numerous roles in expressing different meanings. Therefore, drama is usually staged or performed with the body serving as a significant element of performance.

Reflexivity as Embodiment: The Looking-Glass Body

On the other hand, the body possesses the social self, which correlates all the senses of individuality. Therefore, it is assumed that interactions among individuals are based on reflexivity of the body. As such, the body assumes a looking-glass appearance, especially with regard to the functions of its components. For instance, the eye is believed to play a sociological function through which individuals interact. Mutual glances among individuals serve as significant means of interaction.

Moreover, the observation of bodies enables individuals to interpret the images observed from the imaginary perspective and, this aspect enables individuals to imagine their personal appearance. It also enables individuals to interpret judgment of the perceived appearance, leading to a self-feeling, which is usually expressed as mortification or pride (Waskul & Vannini, 2005). Therefore, bodies appear to be interactively embodied; thus, assuming the looking-glass appearance.

Body as Province of Meaning: The Phenomenological Body

From a phenomenological perspective, the body serves as a province of meaning. The body serves as an instrumental tool for identifying emotional and social order, especially with regard to personal and communal perspective. Sociologists argue that the body forms a fundamental element of social practices. The phenomenological aspect of the body is manifested in the world of art and religious experiences. Imagery, phantasm and dreams portray the body as a province of meaning. Moreover, the child's play word and the forces of insanity exemplify the body as a finite province of meaning. "We have a body that serves as a fundamental corporeal anchor in the world; we also experience ourselves through numerous 'bodies of meaning'" (Waskul & Vannini, 2005). It is believed that the meaning presented by metaphors implies the role of the body, which is manifested in the embodied action; thus, the body can be interpreted appropriately by the frameworks of meaning.

Body as Story: The Narrative Body

Recently, the field of Literature has generated a new theory, which is based on the narrative framework. In the new theory, personhood is perceived as a narrative accomplishment. Narratives are believed to enhance coherence and continuity of personhood because; stories hold persons together. This aspect is enhanced by the presence of syntax, language and grammar of socio-cultural and institutional discourse. Therefore, the narrative body rests in the stories individuals tell about the bodies of other individuals and, this is also evidenced in the culture of beauty.

Body as Trace of Culture: The Socio-Semiotic Body

Semiological conceptualizations portray the body as an instrument for expressing subjectivity to other individuals. From another perspective, the body is perceived to as a source of communication, especially with regard to the understanding of the social interaction that occurs between bodies. However, the socio-semiotic body is usually manifested in the social structure, which is constructed within embodied inequalities.

Sociology of Health, Illness and Sexuality

Sociology of the body has provided a reliable platform for elucidating significant social issues, which are believed to cause challenges of health. Issues such as eating disorders, globalization of food production and decisions on dietary regimes are influenced by social relations. It is believed that women are more prone to eating disorders because; the body image of women is usually skinny compared to a masculine body of men (Gimlin, 2002). In addition, the women body encompasses attractiveness; thus, women are usually judged in regard to their appearance but, not their accomplishments.

In general, the pillars of the sick role define the social aspect of an individual's health. These pillars state that the sick individual is entitled to fundamental rights and privileges; thus, they can withdraw from their responsibilities to regain health. They also state that the onset of a disease does not relate to the individual's behavior. Therefore, the new branch of sociology explains health as part of symbolic interaction, in which it approaches it from the race, gender and social technology perspective. Social classes are also considered being significant determinants of health.

Social classes are believed to define individuals' health. Sociologists argue that, the healthiest countries are those whose income is evenly distributed among their populations. In addition, high levels of social integration contribute significantly to the health of individuals (Bury & Gabe, 2004). Some social aspects such as the level of literacy are believed to influence preventive health behaviors; thus, poorly literate populations are more exposed to health problems than highly literate populations.

In regard to race, the social nature of ethnic groups determines their health status. As a result, some health issues are experienced more often among some ethnic populations than in others. For instance, life expectancy, which serves as a significant demographic factor portrays differences between the black and white races. In 2003, life expectancy for black females was estimated to be 76 years compared to 80 years life expectancy experienced by their white counterparts. There are also significant racial gaps between the whites and blacks and, this is attributable to the differences in their cultural conditions. On the other hand, social demographic factors are also believed to be correlated to the prevalence of some health conditions. In the U.S, hypertension has been found to be highly prevalent among the black men compared to whites.

On the other hand, diet is believed to be one of the significant elements, which distort the body. This is commonly referred to as the social technology, in which dieting is regarded as one of the most powerful tools for altering individuals' bodies. In addition, the phenomenal socialization of nature is determined by social decisions of individuals. Therefore, the essence of reproduction as a natural phenomenon can be regarded to as a social element and, human sexuality can be attributed to social behaviors.

Conclusion

Conclusively, the new branch of sociology highlights the significance of the body by portraying it as a fundamental element of social life. Sociologists have digressed into this field by theorizing the body into physical, personal, political and expressive bodies. On the other hand, this field discusses the body in symbolic interactions extensively to manifest the significance of the body as an instrument of meaning, performance, story and culture. It also relates social behavior with the health of individuals and, unearths diverse perspectives on the aspect of human sexuality.

In general, the sociology of the body reveals the significance of the body as a fundamental element of social life. It portrays the body and mind to be of equal significance because; the body acquires knowledge from the environment and transforms it into physical skills and abilities.

References

Bury, M., & Gabe, J. (2004). *The Sociology of Health and Illness: A Reader.* London, U.K: Routledge.

Gimlin, D. (2002). *Body Work: Beauty and Self-Image in American Culture.* Berkeley, CA: University of California Press.

Haraway, D. (2001). "A Manifesto for Cyborgs." in D. Trend (Ed.), *Reading Digital Culture.* Malden, MA: Blackwell.

Heim, M. (20010. "The Erotic Ontology of Cyberspace." in D. Trend (Ed.), *Reading Digital Culture.* Malden, MA: Blackwell.

Kelland, J. (2006). *Theorizing the Body: Developing a Framework for Understanding the Body in Online Learning Environments.* Retrieved from http://www.adulterc.org/Proceedings/2006/Proceedings/Kelland.pdf

Low, J., & Malacrida, C. (2008). *Sociology of the Body: A Reader.* Oxford, U.K: Oxford University Press.

Shilling, C. (2003). *The Body and Social Theory (second edition).* Thousand Oaks, CA: Sage.

Waskul, D., & Vannini, P. (2005). *Introduction: The Body in Symbolic Interaction.* Retrieved from http://www.ashgate.com/pdf/SamplePages/Body_Embodiment_Intro.pdf

YOUR KNOWLEDGE HAS VALUE

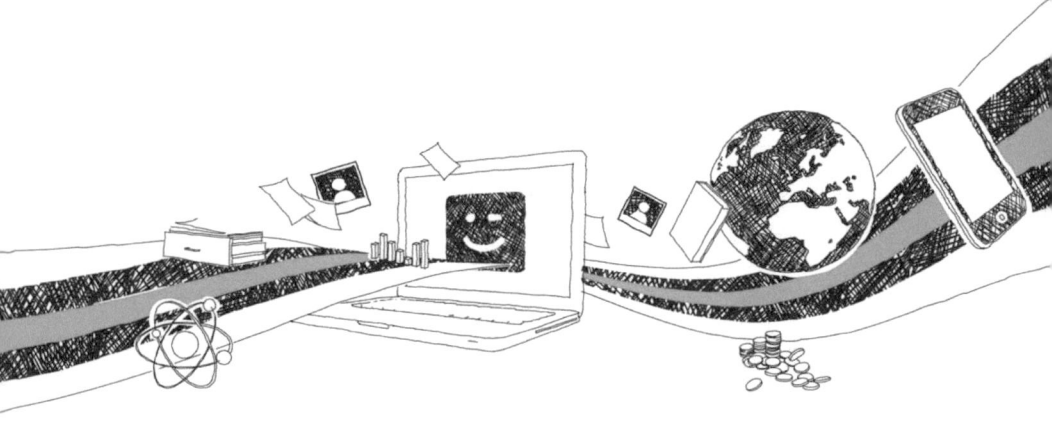

- We will publish your bachelor's and master's thesis, essays and papers

- Your own eBook and book - sold worldwide in all relevant shops

- Earn money with each sale

Upload your text at www.GRIN.com and publish for free